ATRIAL FIBRILLATION DIET

A Beginner's 2-Week Guide on Managing AFib, With Curated Recipes and a Sample Meal Plan

Jeffrey Winzant

mindplusfood

DISCLAIMER

By reading this disclaimer, you are accepting the terms of the disclaimer in full. If you disagree with this disclaimer, please do not read the guide.

All of the content within this guide is provided for informational and educational purposes only, and should not be accepted as independent medical or other professional advice. The author is not a doctor, physician, nurse, mental health provider, or registered nutritionist/dietician. Therefore, using and reading this guide does not establish any form of a physician-patient relationship.

Always consult with a physician or another qualified health provider with any issues or questions you might have regarding any sort of medical condition. Do not ever disregard any qualified professional medical advice or delay seeking that advice because of anything you have read in this guide. The information in this guide is not intended to be any sort of medical advice and should not be used in lieu of any medical advice by a licensed and qualified medical professional.

The information in this guide has been compiled from a variety of known sources. However, the author cannot attest to or guarantee the accuracy of each source and thus should not be held liable for any errors or omissions.

You acknowledge that the publisher of this guide will not be held liable for any loss or damage of any kind incurred as a result of this guide or the reliance on any information provided within this guide. You acknowledge and agree that you assume all risk and responsibility for any action you undertake in response to the information in this guide.

Using this guide does not guarantee any particular result (e.g., weight loss or a cure). By reading this guide, you acknowledge that there are no guarantees to any specific outcome or results you can expect.

All product names, diet plans, or names used in this guide are for identification purposes only and are the property of their respective owners. The use of these names does not imply endorsement. All other trademarks cited herein are the property of their respective owners.

Where applicable, this guide is not intended to be a substitute for the original work of this diet plan and is, at most, a supplement to the original work for this diet plan and never a direct substitute. This guide is a personal expression of the facts of that diet plan.

Where applicable, persons shown in the cover images are stock photography models and the publisher has obtained the rights to use the images through license agreements with third-party stock image companies.

CONTENTS

INTRODUCTION

According to the Centers for Disease Control and Prevention, or the CDC, it is estimated that by 2030, 12.1 million of the US population will have Atrial Fibrillation.

In 2018, almost 15% of the 175,326 deaths pointed out that Atrial Fibrillation was the underlying cause of death.

If you are a part of the population that has this disease, this guide will help you understand more about Atrial Fibrillation and will also provide you with how you can manage your symptoms, which will lead to improving your condition.

According to the National Institutes of Health, or the NIH, Atrial Fibrillation, or AFib, is "one of the most common types of arrhythmias or irregular heart rhythms." It's a heart condition that causes the heart to have irregular and, oftentimes, abnormally fast heart rates.

Even experts aren't entirely sure what causes AFib, but it usually happens when electric impulses abnormally fire up the atria. This causes irregular heartbeats and palpitations, chest pains, and lightheadedness, to name a few.

The risk of this disease increases as the patient gets older. It is also noted that 1 out of 7 strokes is caused by AFib. Thus, it's usually given proper medical attention to alleviate symptoms and improve the condition. In addition to that, you can contribute to this by starting a healthier, heart-friendlier lifestyle, which is what this guide is all about. You'll also learn about the following:

- All about Atrial Fibrillation
- Risk factors of AFib
- Common symptoms and causes
- The Mediterranean Diet
- Two-week guide on starting the diet
- Recipes good for AFib patients

WHAT IS ATRIAL FIBRILLATION?

Atrial Fibrillation is a clinically proven but largely unaddressed cardiovascular disease. Atrial fluid is pumped around the heart by contractions of the walls of blood vessels in the atrium. The heart itself is filled with the trial waste product, or atrial mucous, which causes the heart to work harder than it normally would. When the flow of blood to the atrium is interrupted for any reason, the result is the automatic constriction of the arteries.

Atrial Fibrillation is the automatic pumping of blood from the heart with the assistance of the atrial cavity. Atrial Fibrillation is the most common cause of sudden death in patients with cardiovascular disease. The spasm of the atrial fluid in the atrium can cause sudden, unexpected death. It is the main cause of sudden cardiac arrest (SCA) in coronary artery disease sufferers. Atrial Fibrillation can have several underlying causes. Two of the more common ones are chronic coughs, asthma, chronic sinusitis, allergies, alcohol abuse, and lung disease.

Risk Factors
People who smoke cigarettes have a greater risk of developing atrial fibrillation. Smoking constricts the blood vessels in the

lungs. The increased risk of stroke due to these blood clots is greater for smokers than for nonsmokers. If you develop atrial fibrillation and are a smoker, you should stop smoking immediately and see your doctor. To be on the safe side, don't smoke even if you have been advised by your doctor to do so. By not smoking, you can reduce your risk of getting a hemorrhagic stroke.

Two other risk factors for atrial fibrillation include being of a black race and men having an enlarged heart. Men have enlarged hearts because the ventricles are made larger. They also have a smaller inlet to the lungs and a smaller ventricle. The atria are larger than the vena cava. People suffering from diabetes are at a greater risk of heart attack or heart failure because the control of blood glucose is affected.

Certain risk factors can increase the risk of atrial fibrillation. If you have diabetes, you have an increased risk of suffering from ECD. If you are a smoker, you will have an increased risk of suffering from a stroke. The atria are misaligned or displaced because of the enlargement of the ventricles in your heart. The misalignment of the upper chambers of your heart affects the normal heart rhythm.

COMMON SYMPTOMS OF ATRIAL FIBRILLATION

Many people experience shortness of breath at times, but they don't always know that it is called atrial fibrillation. The majority of people will experience shortness of breath due to many different conditions, which means that the sufferer needs to find out what type of shortness of breath (also known as atrial fibrillation) they have before determining a treatment plan.

These are some of the main symptoms of atrial fibrillation:

• **Shortness of Breath**
Along with a fast heart rate, shortness of breath can be due to many other factors as well. Atrial fibrillar rhythms are caused by many things, such as heart disease, tumors, infections, high blood pressure, stroke, and more. It's important to know if you're experiencing any of these symptoms because many of them could be the symptoms of something more serious. Atrial fibrillar rhythms often happen without causing the sufferer any harm,

but they can still be dangerous if left untreated or not taken care of properly. This is why it's crucial for anyone who experiences shortness of breath or any other irregular heart rhythms to get medical attention as soon as possible.

• Two Upper Chambers

Two upper chambers are needed in the ventricles of the heart for proper blood circulation. However, when atrial fibrillation occurs, there are usually two upper chambers instead of just one. When this occurs, the ventricles aren't able to circulate all of the oxygen-rich blood that they need, which leads to symptoms such as shortness of breath, dizziness, tingling, and numbness in the arms, legs, and even toes. Two upper chamber problems also mean that the ventricles aren't getting the proper amount of oxygen-rich blood.

Other symptoms include:

• Uneasy and rapid heartbeats

Atrial fibrillation is one of the most common conditions that is connected with heart palpitations, which are an abnormality in the rhythm of the heart that can feel like a fluttering or thumping in the chest. Even while these bouts of an irregular heartbeat can be caused by factors such as stress, worry, or the use of certain drugs, it is important not to disregard them since they may signal a more serious underlying issue. Anyone who is experiencing heart palpitations is strongly encouraged to seek the advice of a trained medical practitioner to receive an accurate diagnosis and formulate an effective treatment strategy.

• Chest pain

Atrial fibrillation can cause individuals to suffer a variety of symptoms, one of which is chest discomfort, which can range from a stabbing sensation to a dull ache. It is also possible for it to radiate to other areas of the body, such as the mouth and the arms. Pain in the chest of this nature is the kind that should never be disregarded and should always prompt a trip to the physician, as it might be an early warning sign of a more serious ailment such as a heart attack. If you are suffering any signs of chest discomfort, you should seek immediate medical assistance so that a correct diagnosis can be made and the underlying cause may be treated.

• Fatigue

As a result of the inefficiency of the heart in pumping blood, those who suffer from atrial fibrillation are more prone to develop feelings of weariness. Even if you haven't been engaging in intense or rigorous physical activity before this, you may still have feelings of weariness and weakness as a result of this. Individuals who have atrial fibrillation may find it easier to manage and live with this symptom if they have a better understanding of the relationship between atrial fibrillation and fatigue, as well as identify techniques that are tailored to their specific requirements.

In addition, many cases of atrial fibrillation can lead to anemia, a disease that is defined by low levels of red blood cells, resulting in greater exhaustion and tiredness. Anemia is a condition that is characterized by low levels of red blood cells. Those who are affected by the ailment must thus be aware of the condition's indications and symptoms to be able to take measures that will lessen the influence it has on their lives.

• Lightheadedness

When experiencing symptoms such as lightheadedness or dizziness, it is critical to seek immediate medical assistance. These symptoms may be the result of atrial fibrillation, which is more serious than a mere annoyance. The forceful contractions of the cardiac muscle lead to ineffective pumping of critical nutrients and oxygen, which are two of the most common symptoms that accompany this ailment. Poor circulation and low blood pressure are also two of the most common symptoms that accompany this condition. A qualified medical professional will be able to render a precise diagnosis and devise an effective treatment strategy that will help a patient's health be restored.

• Symptoms of swelling in the lower legs or feet
Edema is the medical term for swelling that can occur in a patient's feet or legs when they have atrial fibrillation. This may be caused by impaired circulation, which leads to fluid accumulation. If you have this symptom, you must make an appointment with a medical professional as soon as possible since it may be an indication of a more serious disease such as congestive heart failure. Because of this, getting an evaluation for these symptoms is necessary if one wants to avoid future difficulties.

• Trouble falling or staying asleep
People who have atrial fibrillation may have a higher risk of developing insomnia, often known as the inability to fall asleep or stay asleep. Concern over the disease may be a big component in these instances; however, it is also possible that the inability to breathe when lying down is the cause of the interrupted sleep cycle. If you are experiencing trouble sleeping, you should seek medical attention as soon as possible since there are therapies available for a wide variety of sleep disorders that can help ease this ongoing problem.

• Changes in the appetite
Alterations in appetite are common in people who have atrial fibrillation. These alterations can range from an increase in hunger as a result of concern about the illness to a reduction in appetite as a result of nausea or vomiting. If you have seen any of these changes in your appetite, you must get medical assistance as soon as possible since these variations may be the result of an underlying disease. After that, medical professionals will be able to assist in the development of the most effective treatment plan

and individualized advice feasible.

If you have had any of the aforementioned symptoms, you must seek medical assistance as soon as you possibly can.

WHAT ARE THE CAUSES?

What are the causes of Atrial Fibrillation? This is a question that you should be asking if you have any knowledge or information on this subject. There are two major reasons for atrial fibrillation; one is due to congenital heart disease and the other is cardiac arrhythmias. When we talk about congenital heart disease, is caused by a defect in the gene that can be passed on only if the mother carries the gene. Some of the defects include small valve structures, enlarged hearts, heart valve disorders, etc. An arrhythmia is caused by either an abnormal heart rhythm or by the excessive pumping of the heart muscles.

Cardiac arrhythmias are considered two upper chambers of the heart that are working abnormally. One of them is called atrial fibrillation. This heart condition is characterized by an irregular pulse pattern, rapid heart rate, and irregular blood pressure. This condition can be life-threatening at times. Atrial fibrillation is often caused by ventricular tachycardia. It is also often associated with ventricular fibrillation.

The irregular heart rate of an atrial fibrillar will make it possible for the atrial cavity to inflate causing the enlargement of the ventricle. This ventricular dysfunction then pumps abnormal blood from the atria to the ventricle. This ventricular dysfunction is commonly caused by two factors, which include the side effect of nitrate salts. Nitrate salts are commonly found in sports drinks and nitrate deficiency at times can cause ventricular fibrillation.

The other cause of atrial fibrillation is ventricular tachycardia. This condition happens when the ventricular rate exceeds a certain level. This condition's main cause is ventricular tachycardia, which makes it impossible for the heart to beat at a normal frequency. The result of ventricular tachycardia is an irregular heart rhythm or cardiomyopathy. This condition has no permanent cure but it can be controlled by using certain medicines.

Obesity is a medical condition that increases the risk of atrial fibrillation. This medical condition occurs when the body mass index is higher than 35%. A large number of obese people suffer from a sleep disorder called sleep apnea. Sleep apnea is a medical condition wherein the individual pauses or stops breathing during sleep. The breathing is obstructed thus the person wakes up sometimes unable to breathe.

Obesity can cause a variety of other medical conditions like hypertension. This condition results in increased pressure in the heart. The heart is unable to pump blood effectively therefore it overworks and becomes stressed. Another medical condition that increases the risk of atrial fibrillation is atherosclerosis in the arteries. This condition occurs when the cholesterol in the blood begins to deposit. Blood vessels are slowly blocked leading to cardiac arrest.

COMPLICATIONS

Atrial fibrillation is a common form of arrhythmia that can have severe health complications if left untreated. The condition is frequently described as being accompanied by symptoms like palpitations, lightheadedness, and chest discomfort. The chance of having a stroke, heart failure, tachycardia-induced cardiomyopathy, and blood clots in the lungs are also associated with atrial fibrillation.

Atrial fibrillation is one of the conditions that can lead to a stroke, which is one of the most dangerous complications since it can cause paralysis or even death if blood supply to different sections of the brain is impeded. This happens when a blood clot develops inside the chambers of your heart and then travels up through your arteries and into your brain, blocking essential vessels that are required for oxygenated blood flow. This can lead to a stroke.

Atrial fibrillation can lead to heart failure owing to inadequate pumping activity, which is produced by inefficient electrical impulses used to transport blood throughout the body during each beat. These signals are utilized to move blood throughout the body during each heartbeat. A person who has edema in their limbs may have symptoms such as shortness of breath, swelling in the feet and ankles, weariness, and weight gain. These symptoms are caused by the buildup of fluid in the limbs.

Tachycardia-Induced Cardiomyopathy is another potential complication of atrial fibrillation which occurs when rapid heart rates prevent adequate time for rest between beats. This can lead to a rapid depletion of protein reserves, which are required for healthy functioning. Cardiomyopathy can be prevented by maintaining a normal resting heart rate. These reserves are then replenished with water, which over time results in an expansion of the heart muscle and weaker contractions while the heart is trying to pump blood throughout the body.

Finally, blood clots in the lungs, also known as pulmonary embolisms, can be extremely dangerous for people who have atrial fibrillation. This condition, which restricts normal movement and function within vital organs such as the lungs, can cause symptoms such as bloody coughing, chest pain, and increased difficulty breathing normally.

Because of the potential risks associated with untreated atrial fibrillation, you should inform your physician of any changes in your physical functioning or levels of energy. This will allow them to determine the appropriate steps for management, which may include alterations to one's way of life or the use of medications, depending on the specific requirements of the individual.

HOW IS ATRIAL FIBRILLATION DIAGNOSED

The most common kind of abnormal heartbeat is called atrial fibrillation. Diagnosis and treatment are necessary to lessen the likelihood of experiencing long-term problems such as a stroke or heart failure. Your doctor could use an electrocardiogram (ECG), echocardiography, an exercise stress test, a Holter monitor, or an Event recorder to identify atrial fibrillation in you. These are just some of the possible tests.

Electrocardiograms, often known as ECGs, are generally the first step in the diagnostic process for atrial fibrillation. To perform an ECG, electrodes are placed on the patient's skin so that the electrical activity in the heart can be measured. The electrocardiogram can offer information on the pace and rhythm of the heart, in addition to any indicators of diseases associated with it.

An echocardiogram is a type of ultrasound examination that generates detailed pictures of the heart by making use of sound waves. It can identify any structural issues with the heart that may be contributing to the symptoms.

The Exercise Stress Test is a diagnostic tool that determines how your body reacts to strenuous physical activity by monitoring your vital signs before, during, and after exercise. This test can identify any changes in heart rate or rhythm that are caused by exercise, and it can also screen for any other possible underlying concerns such as coronary artery disease or valve disorders that could create symptoms that are similar to those that are being exhibited by the patient.

A Holter Monitor is an electrocardiogram (ECG) recording device that is worn for twenty-four to forty-eight hours and monitors continuous ECG recordings over a longer period. It can detect arrhythmias that would not be apparent in a single ECG recording session. An event recorder is another gadget that may be used if you have symptoms that come and go at different times throughout the day. This device can be carried with you at all times and will record the activity of your heart whenever you encounter symptoms.

Your physician will consider the results of all of these tests, as well as a physical exam and study of your medical history, to arrive at a diagnosis of atrial fibrillation, which will allow him or her to devise the most appropriate treatment strategy for you.

MEDICAL TREATMENTS FOR ATRIAL FIBRILLATION DIET

When it comes to the treatment of atrial fibrillation, drugs are frequently required to both controls the rhythm of the heart and lower the risk of potential issues that may arise in the long run. Antiarrhythmic medicines, beta-blockers, calcium channel blockers, and blood thinners are examples of medications that are frequently administered to patients.

To treat irregular cardiac rhythms, antiarrhythmic medicines are often prescribed to patients. They achieve their beneficial effects by interrupting or resetting the abnormal electrical signals in your heart that are responsible for arrhythmias. Drowsiness, lightheadedness, nausea, and headaches are some of the possible adverse effects of this medication.

Atrial fibrillation can be treated with beta-blockers, which not only reduce the heart rhythm but also alleviate some of the symptoms associated with the condition, such as chest discomfort and palpitations. These drugs are effective because they block particular hormones that are the root cause of irregular heartbeat. In addition, they can be used to treat hypertension and a variety of other cardiac disorders. Tiredness, chilly hands, erectile dysfunction, and difficulty sleeping are some of the common adverse effects that may occur.

Calcium channel blockers are medications that are intended to relax the muscles around your heart and expand blood arteries throughout the body. This allows for easier circulation of blood throughout the body. This assists in lowering blood pressure, which in turn lessens the symptoms of atrial fibrillation, such as feeling dizzy or having difficulty breathing. Constipation, nausea, and headaches are some of the potential adverse effects that might occur.

Last but not least, a person who has atrial fibrillation may be given blood thinners or anticoagulants as a prescription to avoid the formation of blood clots, the formation of which raises the chance of having a stroke. These drugs have their therapeutic effect by inhibiting the normal functioning of clotting factors already present in the circulation, while also lowering the activity of additional factors that might contribute to clotting in general. Some of the potential negative effects of this medication include stomach discomfort, nosebleeds, and bleeding gums.

Before you start taking these medications, you and your physician need to have a conversation about the potential risks associated with them. This will allow you to prepare for any adverse reactions or allergies you might experience, and it will also allow you to discuss alternative treatment options if you end up needing them.

MANAGING ATRIAL FIBRILLATION THROUGH LIFESTYLE CHANGES

C hanging your lifestyle to manage atrial fibrillation is an excellent method to help regulate and maybe reduce the frequency of your episodes. Modifications to your lifestyle, such as dietary changes, stress management, and regular exercise, may help regulate your heart rate and reduce the symptoms associated with atrial fibrillation. However, the efficacy of these changes will depend on the specifics of your medical condition.

Alterations to one's eating pattern are a crucial component of treatment for atrial fibrillation. It is possible to enhance one's general health while simultaneously managing arrhythmias by decreasing the amount of salt consumed, increasing the amount of fiber obtained from fruits and vegetables consumed, and keeping saturated fat consumption to a minimum. Because of their anti-inflammatory effects, some foods like onions and garlic may also be effective in the management of atrial fibrillation, according to the findings of some studies.

In addition to maintaining a healthy diet, participating in consistent physical exercise is vital for improving overall health. This is because building stronger muscles surrounding the heart can help minimize the risk of arrhythmias occurring. Because exercise may have an effect on every system in the body, you must consult with your primary care physician before beginning any new exercise routine to determine whether or not it is appropriate for you based on the information included in your medical record.

In addition, methods of stress reduction such as yoga, tai chi, or meditation can assist in the management of symptoms by lowering levels of worry or racing thoughts, both of which, if left unchecked, could result in an atrial fibrillation episode that is more severe.

When coping with atrial fibrillation, it is essential to be aware of the kinds of activities that should be avoided at all costs. Consuming alcohol or caffeine can make existing symptoms worse, and excessive exposure to situations or temperatures that could provoke more severe episodes should be avoided whenever feasible. Drinking alcohol or drinking caffeine can also make existing conditions worse.

In addition, patients should always consult with their doctor before taking any new medications, including those available over-the-counter or as herbal supplements. This is because there is a possibility that new medications will interact negatively with the medications that are already being taken for the treatment of atrial fibrillation.

Overall, it is possible to manage atrial fibrillation through a combination of medication, lifestyle changes, and dietary adjustments that focus on reducing inflammation while simultaneously providing beneficial nutrition to support long-term health goals. These changes can be made to manage atrial fibrillation. If you want to get the most out of your treatment plan, you need to have a conversation with your physician about what options are available to you based on your specific requirements.

THE MEDITERRANEAN DIET

I f you are suffering from the symptoms of atrial fibrillation then you should consider following a Mediterranean diet. Following a healthy diet such as this one will be one of the best decisions you can do to help in managing your condition. The diet has been proven to help lower the risk of atrial fibrillation in many patients.

Just a reminder though, the Mediterranean diet nor the AFib diet is made to cure atrial fibrillation. These diets, although beneficial, only help in managing the symptoms and conditions to help improve the quality of your life. It's still important to consult with your doctor regarding following a diet because you want to make sure that you're not depriving your body of the nutrients it needs to function properly.

If you have been diagnosed with this condition, then it is very important to follow a well-balanced and healthy diet. This can help to improve your overall health. The following foods can be included in a Mediterranean diet as part of effective treatment: eggs, olive oil, fruit, vegetables, legumes, seeds, nuts, and whole grains. If you like to eat these foods then you can use them as a great start to a healthy lifestyle.

Eggs are rich in proteins, which are essential in keeping the body healthy. It is therefore essential to eat plenty of eggs daily, but if you are suffering from heart disease or any other condition, then consuming too many eggs may be counter-productive. To reap maximum benefits from your atrial fibrillation diet, try and eat six small eggs per day. While this does not replace healthy eating, it can be part of a healthy, balanced, and a-fib-reducing diet.

Olive oil is an excellent source of vitamin E and is a great alternative to processed foods. High blood pressure is often believed to be caused by saturated fat, but olive oil contains significantly less fat than the standard oils used in the kitchen. Try to substitute regular butter and animal fat with olive oil whenever possible. High blood pressure can also be reduced through the use of supplements, so research the benefits of taking fish oil, flaxseed oil, and omega-3 supplements.

While the atrial fibrillation diet does not specifically state that you should exclude or include any particular food item, it typically recommends avoiding processed foods as much as possible. Processed foods are generally high in sodium, sugar, saturated fat, salt, and flour. The atrial fibrillation diet recommends eating lean meats, chicken, and fish and consuming as little processed food as possible. The recommended quantities of fish are approximately two ounces for every pound of desired body weight.

While you're on the atrial fibrillation diet, it's important to make sure that you are getting plenty of fiber, as well as water to help your body function properly. Fiber can easily move waste through your digestive tract, which keeps your stomach feeling full. On the other hand, water flushes out toxins that have been built up in your digestive system. The atrial fibrillation diet usually recommends about one teaspoon of fiber per meal, and this can help you feel full and keep your body functioning properly. While you're on the diet, you must drink at least eight glasses of water throughout the day for the best results.

One of the most crucial things that you need to remember while you're on this diet plan is that you need to stay away from grains, potatoes, and most processed foods. Instead, you want to eat more fresh fruits and vegetables and more foods that are cooked in oils like olive oil, coconut oil, sesame oil, and other healthy fats. By eliminating processed foods and incorporating more whole foods and plant-based foods, you will quickly notice a huge difference in how your body feels and behaves. If you're looking to reduce high blood pressure symptoms, you can find many health benefits by following the Atrial Fibrillation Diet.

In detail, here are lists of foods you can use as a guide in updating your meal plans:

Foods to Eat
The foods that fall under this category mainly are fresh produce and foods rich in magnesium, and potassium, healthy fats like unsaturated and polyunsaturated like omega-3, and other foods rich in vitamins and minerals.

- fresh fruits
- blueberries
- cranberries
- raspberries
- strawberries
- avocados
- bananas
- apricots
- oranges
- coconut water
- prunes
- vegetables, except the leafy ones
- tomatoes
- squash

- spinach
- root vegetables, such as sweet potatoes and beets
- whole grains
- brown rice
- quinoa
- oats
- herring
- mackerel
- salmon
- sardines
- tuna
- walnuts
- flaxseed
- avocado
- olive oil
- canola oil
- almonds
- hazelnuts
- cashews
- peanuts and peanut butter
- yogurt

Foods to Avoid

The list below mostly consists of foods that may trigger symptoms and worsen the risks of heart diseases, diabetes, and cholesterol, such as foods rich in trans fat, saturated fat, sodium, and sugar—generally considered junk foods. Depending on your condition, you may be advised to either limit these foods or completely avoid them.

- alcoholic beverages
- caffeine
- tea
- energy drinks
- margarine
- crackers

- cookies
- potato chips
- doughnuts
- butter
- cheese
- red meat
- soda
- sweet baked goods
- fried foods
- processed foods
- food made with partially hydrogenated vegetable oils
- leafy vegetables or rich in vitamin K
- gluten
- grapefruit

In some cases, you must consult with your doctor about changing your diet, as there may be some foods that fall in the to-eat category but may interfere with your medications, thus affecting your overall health. For example, if you're taking blood-thinning medication, you might be advised to refrain from consuming large amounts of leafy green vegetables that are rich in vitamin K. Gluten is also considered a type of food that must be avoided, especially if you have other conditions or are gluten-intolerant.

Foods high in tyramine—a natural compound found in different types of food—as this compound can raise blood pressure and heighten the risk of symptoms for AFib. Tyramine is usually found in:

- aged cheeses
- cured meats, typically treated with salt and/or nitrate
  - dry-type summer sausages
  - pepperoni
  - salami
- kimchi, sauerkraut, and other fermented cabbages
- soy sauce, fish sauce, shrimp sauce, and other particular sauces

- Marmite and other yeast-extract spread
- broad bean pods

Another thing to consider in this diet is the preparation itself, which should mainly be heart-healthy cooking methods. Some of these methods are steaming and poaching fish and vegetables. Baking, roasting, and sauteing are perfect for lean meats.

The American Heart Association, or AHA, recommended the Mediterranean-style diet as it provides a great list of foods that must be emphasized, included, and limited in a meal plan. The Medical News Today created this table that identifies the foods that fall under these categories:

Frequently	vegetables whole grains olive oil fruits legumes
Less frequently	fish chicken and turkey nuts and seeds eggs dairy
Rarely	added sugars highly processed foods fatty, processed meats refined carbohydrates

Sample 7-Day Meal Plan
Starting a new routine will be challenging, that's for sure. When that routine mainly focuses on food, the challenge becomes much more difficult. In an attempt to help you ease into the new diet meal plan, here is a sample 7-day meal plan that you may use or take inspiration from.

Sunday
Breakfast - Muesli-Style Oatmeal
Lunch - Arugula and Mushroom Salad
Dinner - Seafood Stew

Monday
Breakfast - Keto Zucchini Walnut Bread
Lunch - Black Beans With Rice
Dinner - Marinated Tuna Steak

Tuesday
Breakfast - Apple Cinnamon Smash Oatmeal
Lunch - Avocado, Cucumber, and Tomato Salad
Dinner - Chicken and Vegetable Curry

Wednesday
Breakfast - Cherry Coconut Porridge
Lunch - Fennel-Crusted Salmon on White Beans
Dinner - Chicken Broth

Thursday
Breakfast - Berry Blast Oats
Lunch - Stuffed Chicken
Dinner - Couscous Salad with Chickpeas

Friday
Breakfast - Spinach Quiche
Lunch - Turkey Sausage and Arugula Pasta
Dinner - Chicken Salad

Saturday
Breakfast - Instant Polenta with Sesame Seeds
Lunch - Vegetable Broth
Dinner - Almond-Crusted Fish

AFIB GUIDE - WEEK 1

After understanding more about the AFib condition and learning about the Mediterranean diet, you can now start navigating through a 2-week meal plan to help you adjust to this new lifestyle.

As mentioned before, changing your diet will be challenging. There will be times when you might feel tempted to break from your meal plans to eat what you're not supposed to, or worse, feel discouraged to continue your diet. Don't feel pressured or give up so easily. The goal of this two-week plan is to help you slowly adjust to your new lifestyle to help you feel better and become healthier, especially in the long run.

Step 1: Curate a proper food list with your doctor
This will probably be the most important on this list. Atrial fibrillation is not a condition that should be taken lightly, especially if you have other conditions that might worsen when you change your meal plan.

Discuss with your doctors the things you may include in your diet and the things you need to avoid. Better yet, know the reasons why certain foods, ingredients, or condiments may be good or bad for you. This way, you'll be able to curate your meal plans with much ease because you understand why you need to include or remove certain food items from your menu. You may also talk about how you can gradually transition because suddenly changing your diet is also not advisable. This will also give you some time to use up the ingredients you have in your pantry, especially the ones you need to avoid once you start your diet.

Step 2: Start making your meal plans according to your food list and lifestyle
Different people have different lifestyles, which of course reflect different needs. The sample meal plan from the previous chapter only showed three basic meals per day. However, if you are used to eating snacks in between those meals, don't hesitate to add them, just make sure that you're substituting unhealthy snacks with heart-healthy ones.

Take care to incorporate the recommendations provided by your doctor, and if you need to, research more about alternative or organic ingredients you can use to make healthier meals before you replace the stocks you have in your pantry.

You may also want to start keeping a diet diary to keep track of what you eat and how each meal affects you in some ways. This way, you can also see the changes in your weight and mood before starting, during, and at the end of the program. A sample diet diary may look as simple as this:

Current weight: Weight goal:		
Day	Meal/Recipe	Notes
1 - Monday	Breakfast: Keto Zucchini Walnut Bread	(Write about what you like and dislike about this meal; was the quantity enough? Did it make you crave your usual breakfast? Etc.)
	Lunch: Black Beans With Rice	

Step 3: Learn about the heart-healthy ways of preparing your meals

As mentioned before, aside from knowing what food is right for you, you also need to learn how to prepare them so you can make the most of the nutrients you can get from these foods. Try to stay away from frying foods. Learn more about the right ways to poach, steam, roast, blanch, boil, etc.

Step 4: Balance staying active and taking a break

Exercising is very important to maintain and support a healthy lifestyle, especially if you want to regulate your blood pressure and blood sugar. This will be easily achieved by eating healthy and doing exercise. Choose a routine workout that will work best for your lifestyle and condition. Brisk walking is one of the simplest and easiest exercises that provide great results. Even older patients can enjoy this. Exercising also helps relax the mind, which greatly affects the mood and helps in easing up your mind especially in dealing with your condition.

On the other hand, it's also greatly advisable to find ways to relax and take a break. If you're working, make sure to find time to enjoy yourself as well, as a form of reward for your hard work. A visit to the spa is one great option. Going on a brief vacation also is a great way to spend time relaxing. Whatever makes you feel relaxed and comfortable, go and do those things.

Step 5: Quit the bad habits
If you're a smoker and/or an alcohol drinker, consider limiting yourself from doing these habits to
quitting them. The nicotine found in cigarettes is a well-known stimulant of AFib, which increases the heart rate and may start an AFib event.

The same goes for alcohol intake. Before, only heavy drinkers were believed to experience AFib; however, now it is also mentioned that even moderate drinking may cause the same event, especially because not all have the same level of alcohol tolerance. A study published in Canada backs up that information, citing that even moderate drinking—around 1 to 21 drinks in a week for men, and around 1 to 14 drinks in a week for women—can trigger symptoms of AFib.

Seek professional help if you must. Quitting these bad habits completely will surely benefit you, but make sure that you consult with your doctor, especially if you're a chain smoker or alcohol-dependent.

Step 6: Watch what you eat
As you're still transitioning to your new meal plans, it's okay if you end up using an ingredient or two that are part of the food list you need to avoid. However, make sure that you take note of these instances and, as much as possible, the amount you use or consume. This is also where your diary will come in handy.

Also part of your transition to healthy eating is controlling how much you eat. Just because you're eating healthy meals doesn't mean you can binge eat. Remember, anything in excess is bad.

It may start with simple things like splitting meals when you're eating out or preparing small portions of dishes per meal. Using a food scale will also be beneficial for you, especially when you're almost always preparing your meals. This way, you can properly keep track of the measurements of the ingredients you will use in your meals.

Overall, keep in mind that the goal for the first week of this diet plan is for you to start making good habits and getting rid of the bad ones. Don't get discouraged if you fail or get tempted during this week, it's usually inevitable. Don't be too hard on yourself. What you should do in return is to keep doing what you need to do to stick to your goals and stay focused. Don't stress yourself out too much.

AFIB GUIDE - WEEK 2

For the second week, it's better to focus on the changes and improvements you have now achieved after the first week. You are probably more used now to the new meal plans and habits you've started. This week is a great opportunity for you to see how the first week has benefited you, which will surely encourage you as you move on to the second half of this program.

Step 7: Observe changes before and after Week 1

Start your week by jotting down your observations regarding the changes you experienced before and after week 1. You may review the notes you made in your diary. Your goal here is to observe the little changes you experience before and after week 1 of your diet. Don't get discouraged if, for example, you notice little to no difference in your weight. What you should be focusing on is how better you feel after choosing to eat and live right.

You might feel lighter and more energetic. You are probably almost always in a better mood. You don't crave junk food as much, and you even started eating less. Your cholesterol and blood sugar may also show some improvement. These are some of the changes you might experience after a few days of eating healthy. These differ in every person, so just take note of these changes and stay motivated.

Step 8: Stick to stricter meal plans

In your second week, you must be less lenient with the ingredients you use in your meals. Make sure that you stick to the recommended foods and ingredients, so you can fully experience their benefits. Assuming you're more used to the new diet program now, you won't have a hard time fully transitioning to consuming heart-healthy meals. Challenge yourself to try a new healthy meal once in a while to make it exciting.

Step 9: Review your two-week diary and check up with the doctor for an assessment
Once the second week is over, you might want to review your notes in your diary again to see how different week 2 is from week 1. This is also a good time to go back to your doctor for an assessment, so you can have much more detailed information on how this 2-week diet helped you for the better. Make sure to bring your diary or diet notes to be shared with your doctor.

This will also be a good time to curate your meal plans in case you want to continue doing this diet.

Step 10: Consider sticking to the diet
After doing step 9, you might be able to have a clearer vision of how these heart-friendly changes help you feel better about yourself, and most especially about your health. If you want to continue doing this diet, all the better. If you feel good about it, why stop doing it?

Your AFib won't go away anytime soon, so the best thing you can do is manage your condition and your symptoms by doing what's best for your body, sticking to those things that benefit you well, especially in the long run.

SAMPLE RECIPES

Arugula and Mushroom Salad

Ingredients:
- 5 oz. arugula washed
- 1 lb. fresh mushrooms
- 1/4 tsp. shoyu
- 1/2 red onion
- 1 tbsp. olive oil
- 1 tbsp. mirin

For tofu cheese:
- 1/8 cup umeboshi vinegar
- 1/2 firm tofu

Instructions:
1. In a bowl, add the rinsed tofu. Crumble and pour in vinegar.
2. In a separate bowl add shoyu, red onions, salt, olive oil, and mirin. 3. Mix to combine.
4. Add in the arugula and toss to combine with the dressing.
5. Serve and enjoy.

Avocado, Cucumber, and Tomato Salad

Ingredients:
- 1/4 cup extra-virgin olive oil
- 1 pc. lemon, juiced
- 1/4 tsp. cumin, ground
- salt, to taste
- freshly ground black pepper, to taste
- 3 medium avocados, cubed
- 1-pint cherry tomatoes, halved
- 1 small cucumber, sliced into half-moons
- 1/3 cup corn
- 2 tbsp. cilantro, chopped

Instructions:
1. Combine avocados, cilantro, corn, cucumber, jalapeño, and tomatoes in a large bowl.
2. In a separate small container, whisk together lemon juice, cumin, and oil to make the salad dressing.
3. Season the dressing with salt and pepper.
4. Toss the salad gently while adding the dressing.
5. Serve immediately.

Chicken Salad

Ingredients:
- 1 small can of premium chunk chicken breast packed in water
- 1 stalk celery, large, finely chopped
- 1/4 cup reduced-fat mayonnaise
- 4 romaine leaves or red leaf lettuce, washed and trimmed
- 2 oz. blue cheese, crumbled
- 8 pcs. cherry tomatoes or 1 ripe tomato, quartered
- 1 cucumber, small and sliced thinly

Instructions:
1. Drain canned chicken and transfer to a bowl.
2. Put in celery and mayonnaise.
3. Mix lightly. Don't crush the chicken.
4. In a separate shallow bowl, place the lettuce neatly.
5. Add the chicken salad in the middle and sprinkle blue cheese over it.
6. Add tomatoes and cucumber slices to the plate.
7. Refrigerate before serving, cover with plastic wrap.

Egg Salad with Avocados

Ingredients:
- 3 medium-sized avocados
- 6 eggs, large and hard-boiled
- 1/3 red onion, medium size
- 3 celery ribs
- 4 tbsps. mayonnaise
- 2 tbsps. freshly squeezed lime juice
- 2 tsp. brown mustard
- 1/2 tsp. cumin powder
- 1 tsp. hot sauce
- salt
- pepper

Instructions:
1. Chop the eggs, celery, and onion.
2. Set aside the avocados, then combine the rest of the ingredients.
3. Slice the avocado in half to take out the pit.
4. Stuff the avocado by spooning the egg salad on its cage.
5. Serve and enjoy.

Vegetable Broth

Ingredients:
- 1 tbsp. oil
- 2 leeks, sliced
- 2 carrots, sliced
- 2 ribs of celery
- 1/4 tsp. salt
- 8 cups water

To make the soup:
- 1 tbsp. oil
- 2 cups potatoes, diced
- 1 cup mushrooms, diced
- 1-1/2 cups cauliflower, diced
- 1 cup onion, diced
- 1 cup celery, diced
- 1 cup carrot, diced
- 1-1/2 cups red beans, cooked
- 2 sprigs of rosemary
- 4 sprigs of thyme
- 2 cups spinach

Instructions:
1. To a pot on medium heat, add oil and leeks.
2. Cook for about three minutes or until they start to soften up.
3. Add carrots and top a few celery stalks with leaves.
4. Cover with water.
5. Add salt. Bring to a simmer and cook until carrots are very tender but not mushy.
6. Turn off the heat and let it cool down a little.
7. When the broth has cooled down, strain out the veggies.
8. Remove carrots and set them aside.
9. Squeeze most of the liquid out of the leeks and celery.

To cook the soup:
1. Add carrots to some of the broth and blend.

2. With a pot on medium heat, add oil, onions, raw carrots, and celery. Cook until onions are translucent, approximately 3 to 5 minutes.

3. Add broth, potatoes, and herbs.

4. Bring to a simmer and cook for 10 minutes.

5. Add cauliflower and red beans.

6. Simmer for another 5 minutes.

7. Add the package of frozen green beans and cook until the potatoes and cauliflower are tender, approximately for another 5 minutes.

8. At the end of cooking, add spinach.

9. Serve warm.

Salmon and Asparagus

Ingredients:
- 2 salmon filets
- 14-oz. young potatoes
- 8 asparagus spears, trimmed and halved
- 2 handfuls cherry tomatoes
- 1 handful of basil leaves
- 2 tbsp. extra-virgin olive oil
- 1 tbsp. balsamic vinegar

Instructions:
1. Heat oven to 428°F.
2. Arrange potatoes into a baking dish.
3. Drizzle potatoes with extra-virgin olive oil.
4. Roast potatoes until they have turned golden brown.
5. Place asparagus into the baking dish together with the potatoes.
6. Roast in the oven for 15 minutes.
7. Arrange cherry tomatoes and salmon among the vegetables.
8. Drizzle with balsamic vinegar and the remaining olive oil.
9. Roast until the salmon is cooked.
10. Throw in basil leaves before transferring everything to a serving dish.
11. Serve while hot.

Seafood Stew

Ingredients:
- 2 tsp. extra-virgin olive oil
- 1 cut bulb fennel
- 2 stalks of celery, chopped
- 2 cups white wine
- 1 tbsp. chopped thyme
- 1 cup chopped shallots
- 6 ounces of shrimp
- 6 ounces of sea scallops
- 1/4 tsp. salt
- 1 cup chopped parsley
- 6 oz. Arctic char
- 2-1/2 cups of water

Instructions:
1. Heat a frying pan on the lowest setting. Add a small amount of oil.
2. Cook the celery, shallots, and fennel for approximately 6 minutes.
3. Pour the wine, water, and thyme into the frying pan.
4. Wait for 10 minutes and allow it to cook.
5. Once much of the water has evaporated, add in the remaining ingredients, and wait for 2 minutes before removing it from the stove.
6. Serve and enjoy immediately.

Lemon-Baked Salmon

Ingredients:
- 2 pcs. lemons, thinly sliced
- 3 lbs. salmon filet
- kosher salt
- black pepper, freshly ground
- 6 tbsp. butter, melted, 6 tbsp.
- 2 tbsp. honey
- 3 cloves garlic, minced
- 1 tsp. thyme leaves, chopped
- 1 tsp. dried oregano
- fresh parsley, chopped, for garnish

Instructions:
1. Preheat the oven to 350°F.
2. Line a rimmed baking sheet with foil. Grease with cooking oil spray.
3. Lay lemon slices on the center of the foil.
4. Season salmon filets on both sides with kosher salt and freshly ground black pepper.
5. Place the filet on top of the lemon slices.
6. Whisk together oregano, thyme, garlic, honey, and butter in a small bowl.
7. Pour the mixture over the salmon filet.
8. Fold the foil up and around the salmon to form a packet.
9. Bake for 25 minutes or until the salmon is cooked through.
10. Switch to broil and continue cooking for 2 more minutes.
11. Garnish with chopped fresh parsley and serve hot.

Marinated Tuna Steak

Ingredients:
- 4 slices tuna steak
- 1/3 cup soy sauce
- 1 tbsp. cider vinegar
- 3 tbsp. olive oil
- 2 tbsp. chopped parsley
- 1 tbsp. chopped rosemary
- 1/2 tsp. chopped oregano
- 1/8 tsp. garlic powder

Instructions:
1. Put together olive oil, soy sauce, parsley, cider vinegar, rosemary, and oregano in a bowl. Mix well to create a marinade mixture.
2. Using a gallon plastic bag, put tuna steaks and marinade mixture. Allow the mixture to coat the tuna by turning the bag over.
3. Leave inside the refrigerator for 30 minutes.
4. Put a small amount of oil on the grill grate. Cook tuna for about 5 minutes per side.
5. Put some of the remaining marinade mixtures on the tuna every few minutes.

Chicken Broth

Ingredients:
- 1 chicken carcass from a leftover roast chicken or bones
- 2 cloves of garlic
- water
- Optional: carrot or parsnip tops, leftover vegetable peelings, and herbs

Instructions:
1. Cover chicken bones with water, whether cooking in a large stockpot, a pressure cooker, or a slow cooker.
2. For the slow cooker, cook on high for 4 hours.
3. For the pressure cooker, set it to cook for an hour.
4. For the stockpot, set it on a low simmer for 3 to 4 hours.
5. Once the time is up, strain the liquid from the broth through a sieve into a large bowl or container.
6. Discard the bones and garlic.
7. Keep the liquid, and pour it into a container.

Stuffed Chicken

Ingredients:
- 4 pcs. chicken breast filets, skinless and boneless
- 1/4 cup feta cheese, crumbled
- 1/4 cup artichoke hearts, finely chopped, drained, and marinated
- 2 tbsp. red peppers, finely chopped, drained, and roasted
- 2 tbsp. green onion, thinly sliced
- 2 tsp. fresh oregano, or 1/2 tsp. if using dried oregano
- 1 tsp. kosher salt
- 1/4 tsp. ground black pepper

Instructions:
1. Cut a pocket in each chicken breast using a sharp knife. Cut through the thickest portion horizontally without cutting through the opposite side.
2. Combine the feta, roasted peppers, artichoke hearts, oregano, and green onions into a mixture.
3. Fill each pocket of the chicken breast with the mixture.
4. Close the opening of the pockets with a wooden toothpick.
5. Season the chicken breast with salt and pepper.
6. Preheat a non-stick large skillet on medium heat.
7. Coat it with cooking spray.
8. Fry the chicken for 10 to 12 minutes on each side, or until the internal temperature reaches at least 165°F.
9. Serve hot.

CONCLUSION

A trial fibrillation, often known as AFib, is a significant medical disorder that, if left untreated, can have catastrophic consequences throughout a person's lifetime. Such who live with atrial fibrillation (AFib) should make significant alterations to their lifestyles, including nutrition and stress management, to better control bouts of the condition and cut down on the frequency of those episodes.

When it comes to the treatment of atrial fibrillation, diet plays an especially significant role. It is possible to enhance one's general health while simultaneously managing arrhythmias by decreasing the amount of salt consumed, increasing the amount of fiber obtained from fruits and vegetables consumed, and keeping saturated fat consumption to a minimum.

Certain research shows that certain foods, such as onions and garlic, exhibit anti-inflammatory characteristics, which may help to alleviate symptoms related to the illness. This makes these foods potential candidates for the category of foods that may be good for AFib patients.

In addition to maintaining a healthy diet, participating in consistent physical exercise is vital for improving overall health. This is because building stronger muscles surrounding the heart can help minimize the risk of arrhythmias occurring. Because exercise can affect any of the body's systems, it is critical to have a conversation with your primary care provider before beginning a new exercise routine.

This will allow you to determine whether or not the new routine is appropriate for you in light of your specific health requirements. In addition, methods of stress reduction such as yoga, tai chi, or meditation can assist in the management of symptoms by lowering levels of worry or racing thoughts, both of which, if left unchecked, could result in an atrial fibrillation episode that is more severe.

Overall, it is possible to manage atrial fibrillation through a combination of medication, lifestyle changes, and dietary adjustments that focus on reducing inflammation while simultaneously providing beneficial nutrition to support long-term health goals. These changes can be made to manage atrial fibrillation. If you want to get the most out of your treatment plan, you need to have a conversation with your physician about what options are available to you based on your specific requirements.

People who live with atrial fibrillation can take steps toward living longer lives free from the debilitating symptoms that are associated with episodes of atrial fibrillation if they receive the appropriate guidance from a healthcare professional and adhere to lifestyle modifications that are designed specifically for people who suffer from atrial fibrillation.

FAQS

1. What is atrial fibrillation?

Atrial fibrillation, also known as AFib, is a type of heart arrhythmia. This means that the heart's electrical system is not working properly, causing the heart to beat in an irregular pattern. AFib is the most common type of arrhythmia, and it affects millions of people worldwide.

2. What are the symptoms of atrial fibrillation?

The most common symptom of AFib is heart palpitations, which are feelings of skipped or extra heartbeats. Other symptoms may include shortness of breath, chest pain, fatigue, and dizziness.

3. What causes atrial fibrillation?

There are many possible causes of AFib, including underlying heart conditions, high blood pressure, diabetes, thyroid problems, sleep apnea, and certain medications. In some cases, the exact cause of AFib cannot be determined.

4. How is atrial fibrillation diagnosed?

AFib is typically diagnosed with a physical exam and a review of your medical history. Your doctor may also order tests such as an electrocardiogram (ECG) or echocardiogram to confirm the diagnosis.

5. How is atrial fibrillation treated?

Treatment for AFib will vary depending on the severity of your symptoms and the underlying cause of your arrhythmia. In some cases, no treatment may be necessary. However, if AFib is causing symptoms or increasing your risk for stroke, you may be prescribed medication or undergo a procedure to restore normal heart rhythm.

6. What are the risks associated with atrial fibrillation?
The main risk associated with AFib is stroke. When the heart beats irregularly, blood can pool in the chambers and form clots. If a clot breaks loose and travels to the brain, it can cause a stroke. Other risks associated with AFib include heart failure and sudden cardiac death.

7. Can atrial fibrillation be prevented?
There is no sure way to prevent AFib, but there are some lifestyle changes that may help lower your risk. These include eating a healthy diet, exercising regularly, managing stress levels, and avoiding smoking and excessive alcohol consumption. If you have an underlying health condition that increases your risk for AFib, controlling this condition can help reduce your risk of developing arrhythmia.

8. What are the long-term effects of atrial fibrillation?
If left untreated, AFib can lead to serious complications such as stroke or heart failure. Therefore, it is important to seek treatment if you are experiencing any symptoms of arrhythmia. With proper treatment and management, most people with AFib can live long and healthy lives

REFERENCES

Amponsah, M. K. D., Benjamin, E. J., & Magnani, J. W. (2013). Atrial fibrillation and race – a contemporary review. Current Cardiovascular Risk Reports, 7(5), 336–345. https://doi.org/10.1007/s12170-013-0327-8.

Atrial fibrillation - what is atrial fibrillation? | NHLBI, NIH. (n.d.). Retrieved January 20, 2023, from https://www.nhlbi.nih.gov/health/atrial-fibrillation.

Atrial fibrillation. (2017, October 20). NHS.UK. https://www.nhs.uk/conditions/atrial-fibrillation/.

Best diet for AFib: Foods to eat and to avoid. (2020, June 30). https://www.medicalnewstoday.com/articles/afib-diet.

CDC. (2022, July 12). Atrial Fibrillation | cdc.gov. Centers for Disease Control and Prevention. https://www.cdc.gov/heartdisease/atrial_fibrillation.htm.

Chen, M. L., Parikh, N. S., Merkler, A. E., Kleindorfer, D. O., Bhave, P. D., Levitan, E. B., Soliman, E. Z., & Kamel, H. (2019). Risk of atrial fibrillation in black versus white medicare beneficiaries with implanted cardiac devices. Journal of the American Heart Association, 8(4), e010661. https://doi.org/10.1161/JAHA.118.010661.

Diet and atrial fibrillation: Should your diet change? (n.d.). Mayo Clinic. Retrieved September 2, 2022, from https://www.mayoclinic.org/diseases-conditions/atrial-fibrillation/expert-answers/diet-atrial-fibrillation/faq-20118479.

Dos and don'ts for eating well with afib—Atrial fibrillation center—Everyday health. (n.d.). EverydayHealth.Com. Retrieved September 2, 2022, from https://www.everydayhealth.com/hs/atrial-fibrillation-management/diet-dos-and-donts/.

Foods to avoid with atrial fibrillation. (2020, July 15). Healthline. https://www.healthline.com/health/atrial-fibrillation/foods-to-avoid.

Liang, Y., Mente, A., Yusuf, S., Gao, P., Sleight, P., Zhu, J., Fagard, R., Lonn, E., & Teo, K. K. (2012). Alcohol consumption and the risk of incident atrial fibrillation among people with cardiovascular disease. Canadian Medical Association Journal, 184(16), E857–E866. https://doi.org/10.1503/cmaj.120412.

Lifestyle changes to manage afib better. (2014, March 18). Healthline. https://www.healthline.com/health/atrial-fibrillation/lifestyle-changes.

Lifestyle strategies for atrial fibrillation(Afib or af). (n.d.). www.heart.org. Retrieved September 2, 2022, from https://www.heart.org/en/health-topics/atrial-fibrillation/treatment-and-prevention-of-atrial-fibrillation/prevention-strategies-for-atrial-fibrillation-afib-or-af.

What is the Mediterranean diet? (n.d.). Www.Heart.Org. Retrieved September 2, 2022, from https://www.heart.org/en/healthy-living/healthy-eating/eat-smart/nutrition-basics/mediterranean-diet.

What to eat to manage atrial fibrillation. (2019, March 7).

Cleveland Clinic. https://health.clevelandclinic.org/managing-your-atrial-fibrillation-what-to-eat-and-avoid/.